Ultimate Sirtfood Diet

Beginners guide for a rapid weight loss to live a long and healthy life. Including Tasty recipes to start in the easiest way

Lisa T. Oliver

© Copyright 2021 All rights reserved.

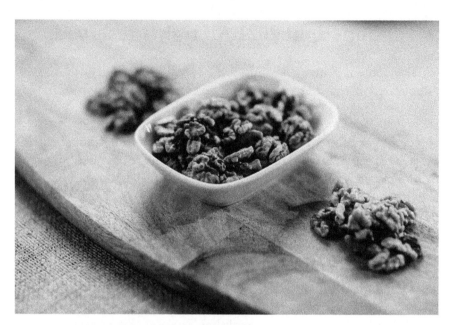

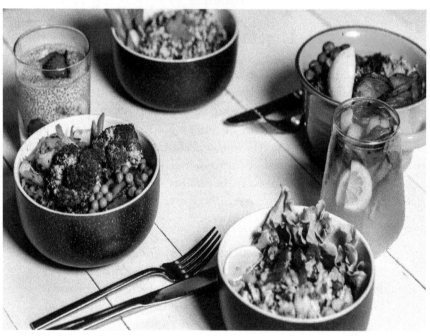

Table Of Contents

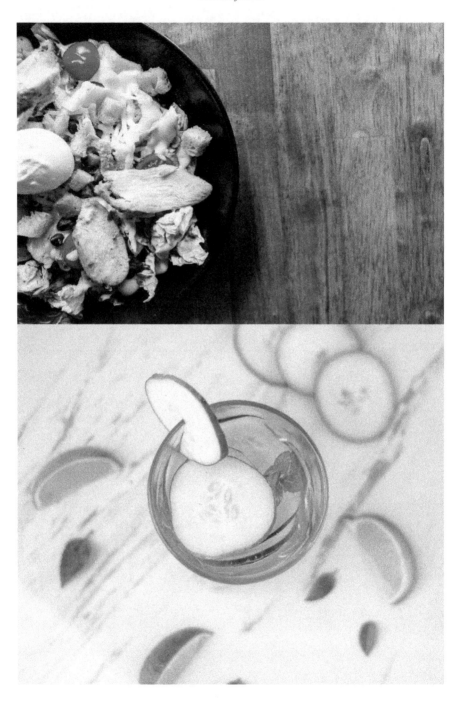

Introduction

The Sirtfood Diet, launched in 2016, has been a trending topic for a while now, with people following the diet very strictly. The creators of the diet suggest that these foods function by activating proteins in the body, referred to as sirtuins. The idea is that sirtuins protect body cells from dying when subjected to stress and regulate metabolism, inflammation, and aging. Sirtuins also boost the body's metabolism and affect its ability to burn fat, providing a weight loss of about seven pounds in a week while retaining muscle. Nonetheless, experts believe that this is solely about fat loss rather than differences in glycogen storage from the liver and skeletal muscle. This diet was developed by UK-based nutritionists, both with MAs in nutritional medicine, and has since gained popularity among athletes and celebrities. Adele and Pippa Middleton are two celebrities who have followed the Sirtfood Diet, and it yielded great results for them. The Sirtfood Diet, like most diets, promotes sustained and significant weight loss, improved health, and better energy. What is it about this diet? Is it just a fad, or is there more to it? Does science back it up? All these questions and more will be answered as you read on. The word "sirt" comes from sirtuins, a group of Silent Information Regulator (SIR) proteins. They boost metabolism, improve muscle efficiency, reduce inflammation, and start the process of fat loss and cell repair. These sirtuins make us healthier, fit, and also help in fighting diseases. Exercise and restrictions on calorie consumption improve sirtuin production in the body.

What Are Sirtfoods?

Sirtuins refer to a protein class that has been proven to regulate the metabolism of fat and glucose. According to research, sirtuins also have a significant impact on aging, inflammation, and cell death.

By consuming foods rich in sirtuins like cocoa, kale, and parsley, you stimulate your skinny gene pathway and lose fat faster.

About the Sirtfood Diet

The Sirtfood Diet plan considers that some foods activate your "skinny gene" and can make you lose about seven pounds in about a week.Certain foods, such as dark chocolate, kale, and wine, contain polyphenols, a natural chemical that imitates exercise and fasting and affects the body. Other sirtfoods include cinnamon, red onions, and turmeric.

The Premise of the Sirtfood Diet The premise of the Sirtfood Diet states that certain foods can mimic the benefits of fasting and caloric restrictions by activating sirtuins, which are proteins in the body. They range from SIRT1 to SIRT7, switch genes on and off, maintain biological pathways, and protect cells from age-related decline. Although intense calorie restriction and fasting are severe, the Sirtfood Diet inventors developed a plan with a focus on eating plenty of sirtfoods. It's a more natural way to stimulate sirtuin genes in the body, also known as skinny genes. In the process, it improves health and boosts weight loss. If you want to start the Sirtfood Diet, planning is required, and access to the ingredients needed to follow the diet correctly.

CHAPTER 1:

Breakfast

1.   Strawberry & Citrus Blend

Preparation time: 30 min

Cooking time: 0 min Servings: 1

Ingredients

75g (3oz) strawberries

One apple, cored

One orange, peeled

½ avocado, peeled and de-stoned

½ teaspoon matcha powder

Juice of 1 lime

Directions:

Place all of the ingredients into a blender with enough water to cover them and process until smooth.

Nutrition:Energy (calories): 290 kcal Protein: 3.17 g Fat: 15.3 g

Carbohydrates: 43.18 g

2.   Grapefruit & Celery Blast

Preparation time: 30 min

Cooking time: 0 min

Servings: 1

Ingredients

One grapefruit, peeled

Two stalks of celery

50g (2oz) kale

½ teaspoon matcha powder

Directions:

Place all the ingredients into a blender with enough water to cover them and blitz until smooth.

Nutrition:

Energy (calories): 27 kcal

Protein: 2.26 g Fat: 0.49 g

Carbohydrates: 4.88 g

3.   Orange & Celery Crush

Preparation time: 30 min

Cooking time: 0 min

Servings: 1

Ingredients

One carrot, peeled

Three stalks of celery

One orange, peeled

½ teaspoon matcha powder

Juice of 1 lime

Directions:

Place all of the ingredients into a blender with enough water to cover them and blitz until smooth.

4.   Tropical Chocolate Delight

Preparation time: 30 min

Cooking time: 0 min

Servings: 1

Ingredients

1 mango, peeled & de-stoned

75g (3oz) fresh pineapple, chopped

50g (2oz) kale

25g (1oz) rocket

1 tablespoon 100% cocoa powder or cacao nibs

150mls (5fl oz.) coconut milk

Directions:

Place all of the ingredients into a blender and blitz until smooth. You can add a little water if it seems too thick.

Nutrition:

Energy (calories): 81 kcal

Protein: 3.43 g

Fat: 1.23 g

Carbohydrates: 19.3 g

5.   Walnut & Spiced Apple Tonic

Preparation time: 30 min

Cooking time: 0 min

Servings: 1

Ingredients

Six walnuts halves

One apple, cored

One banana

½ teaspoon matcha powder

½ teaspoon cinnamon

Pinch of ground nutmeg

Directions:

Place all of the ingredients into a blender and add sufficient water to cover them.

Blitz until smooth and creamy

Nutrition:

Energy (calories): 284 kcal

Protein: 4.85 g Fat: 18.85 g

Carbohydrates: 30.08 g

6.   Pineapple & Cucumber Smoothie

Preparation time: 30 min

Cooking time: 0 min

Servings: 1

Ingredients

50g (2oz) cucumber

One stalk of celery

Two slices of fresh pineapple

Two sprigs of parsley

½ teaspoon matcha powder

A squeeze of lemon juice

Directions:

Place all of the ingredients into the blender with enough water to cover them and blitz until smooth.

Nutrition:

Energy (calories): 416 kcal

Protein: 4.44 g Fat: 18.31 g

Carbohydrates: 61.05 g

7.   King Prawn Fry Almond Noodles

Preparation Time: 10 minutes

Cooking Time: 30 minutes

Servings: 4

Ingredients

300 grams Buckwheat / Soba Noodles When you try to get 100% buckwheat, you can

Two tablespoons extra virgin vegetable oil

cut1 purple onion sliced thin

Two celery chopped 2 Stick chopped

100g bananas approximately

100g green beans cut 33cm

ginger grated

Three garlic cloves grated or finely chopped

One germander speedwell by removing chili seeds/membrane and finely chopped (or taste)

600 Gram Raja Prawns tablespoons parcel two tablespoons Tamari / Soybean cut 2(or if you like) " will get it!)

Directions:

Cook the noodles for 3-5 minutes or until they are your liking. Drain, rinse in cold water. Drizzle over a touch of vegetable oil, mix and set aside.

While the noodles are cooking, prep the remaining ingredients.

In a skillet or large fry pan, fry the purple onions and celery over a little vegetable oil over a yellow onion until softened for 3 minutes, then add the bananas and green beans and cook medium-high heat for 3 minutes.

Heat again and add ginger, garlic, chili, and prawns. Fry for 2-3 minutes until the prawns hot all the way through.

Add the noodles, tamari/soy sauce, and cook for 1 minute until the noodles hot again. Sprinkle with parsley and serve.

8.   Sautéed Mushroom Gouda And Kale Potato Skins

Preparation Time: 10 minutes

Cooking Time: 60 minutes

Servings: 4

Ingredients

6 (or three as a hearty main) as a side

mushrooms

1 tbsp. butter

1 tbsp. vegetable oil

One small onion, finely chopped

Eight white buttons (Ceremony) mushrooms,

One clove garlic, minced.

One teaspoon thyme

wine cup wine or broth

salt and pepper taste

Potatoes

Six red Idaho potatoes or three russet potatoes

Two tablespoons vegetable oil, split

One tablespoon butter

cream

sour cup sour co cup parcels Grated gouda (or cheddar, gruyere, Or comet)

Keel. Banana paste

1 bunch (approx. / Lb. / 226 gr), de-steamed and coarsely chopped

One clove, peel

⅓ cup nut

juice lemon

22 tbsp. Parmesan-Reggiano cheese, grated

2 tbsp. Romano cheese, grated tsp.

3Spoon Extra-Virgin Vegetable Oil

ions cup cooking water, plus if necessary

Directions:

Mushrooms

Melt butter with oil in a pan over medium-high heat. Add onion and sauce, until translucent, about 6 7 minutes.

Add garlic and thyme and fragrant for a few minutes.

Add chopped Ceremony mushrooms and sauté 'until they turn golden brown and begin caramel for about 10 minutes.

Add the wine (or broth), stir the pan, and cook until most of the liquid has evaporated, about 3 minutes.

Season with salt and pepper, add parsley and take away from heat. Cancel.

Potato

Preheat the oven to 400 ° F (200 ° C) and place a rack in the middle.

Gently rub the potatoes, but do not peel. Pierce several times with a fork. Place on an external baking sheet and bake for 25 half an hour (40 minutes if you are using red potatoes).

When they are handled cool enough, slice the potatoes in half, scoop out most of the meat but leave a touch attached to the skin to aid them in holding their shape (leave about ¼ inch of skin and potatoes.)

Melt butter and mix with vegetable oil. Brush the skin and outer part of the skin and bake the skin for an additional 5–10 minutes until it was well and crispy.

Kale Pesto

Bring a heavy salty pot of water to a boiling boil. Add garlic and banana (bound submerge it underwater) and blanch for 3 minutes.

Using a slotted spoonful of fish, take out the banana and garlic from the water and transfer a colander. Allow cool slightly and squeeze several glasses of water on the back of the spoon (or use your hands if you dare).

Add walnuts to a kitchen appliance; the lentils are mixed until the mixture turns into a coarse meal. Add fennel, garlic, and juice.

Pulse until choppy and almost smooth.

I employ the spatula, lowering the edges: Throat-in Parmesan Cheese, Romano Cheese, and Cayenne Flakes (if using). Pulse again, and while the kitchen appliance slowly moving, add water until the peaches a creamy consistency. Transfer the black paste to a bowl and employ a spoonful stirring within the vegetable oil until it is completely absorbed.

If the banana passbooks too thick, add more water (not oil) up a teaspoon at a time until it reaches the specified consistency

Gather the pot skins in a large bowl mash the Potato flesh until it forms a sticking mass. Add sour cream, cup gouda, banana peso (I used about four tablespoons), and season with salt and pepper.

Stuffing filling within prepared pot peels, top with mushrooms, and sprinkle with remaining odd cup Gouda.

Pop in the oven for about 15 to twenty minutes finish.

9.   Steak And Balsamic Vinaigrette With Strawberry Arugula Salad

Preparation Time: 10 minutes

Cooking Time: 30 minutes

Servings: 4

Ingredients

Steak

4 Steak of your choice (Beef Tenderloin picture)

Steak Spice (Montreal Steak Spice was used in the photos)

1 Tbsp. Oil

Salad

6 cups Arugula

6 oz. Raspberry (1 cup)

6 oz. Blueberries (1 cup)

1 cup strawberries (chopped)

1/2 cup feta cheese (crumbled)

1/4 cup diluted almonds

balsamic vinaigrette

1/4 cup balsamic vinegar

1/4 cup vegetable oil

Three tablespoons sugar

1 / 2 tablespoons Dijon mustard

Salt and pepper.Directions:

Steak:

Season steak and allow it to sit at temperature for 5-10 minutes.

Heat the oil during a cast-iron skeleton over medium-high heat. Wait until the oil boiling; it will flicker.

Add steak to the pan, do not touch it. Cook for five minutes, flip over, and cook for 3 minutes or until the internal temperature reaches 130–135 ° F (for medium-rare).

Transfer the steak to a plate and allow it to rest for five minutes before cutting into strips.

Salad

While the steak relaxes, combine all the salad ingredients in a large bowl.

Stir all the vinaigrette ingredients together during a small shaker, then add a salad and toss coat evenly.

Serve, but.

Divide salad in4 bowls and top with steak.

CHAPTER 2:

Lunch

10.   Spicy SpareRibs With Roasted Pumpkin

Preparation time: 10 minutes

Cooking time: 25 minutes

Servings: 4

Ingredients:

400g pork ribs

A spoon of coconut amino acids

Honey spoon

A scoop of olive oil

50 g shallots

Garlic clove

Green paper

One slice onion

One red pepper

One red pepper

For the roasted pumpkin:

One slice of pumpkin

One tablespoon coconut oil

a teaspoon of chili powder:

Directions:

Pickled pork ribs the day before yesterday.

Cut the ribs into four small pieces: mix coconut amino acids, honey, and olive oil in a bowl. Chopped green onions, garlic, and peppers, then add. Spread the ribs on the plastic container and pour the marinade. Place them in the refrigerator overnight.

Cut onions, peppers, and peppers into small pieces and place in a slow cooker. Spare ribs (including marinade) and cook for at least 4 hours.

Preheat the pumpkin to 200 ° C.

Cut the pumpkin on the moon and place it on a baking sheet lined with parchment paper.

Place a spoonful of coconut oil on the baking sheet and season with chili, pepper, and salt. Roast the pumpkin in the oven for about 20 minutes, and then serve it with the ribs.

11. Roast Beef With Grilled Vegetables

Preparation time: 10 minutes

Cooking time: 55 minutes

Servings: 4

Ingredients:

500 g roast beef

Garlic clove (squeezed)

One teaspoon fresh rosemary

400 g broccoli

200g carrots

400 g zucchini

a spoonful of olive oil

Directions:

Rub roast beef with sweet pepper, salt, garlic, and rosemary.

Heat the pan over high heat and fry the meat for about 20 minutes, or until brown spots appear on all flesh sides.

Then wrap it with aluminum foil and let it sit for a while.

Before serving, slice the roast beef into thin slices.

Preheat the oven to 205 ° C. Put all the vegetables in the pan.

Season the vegetables with a little olive oil and then season with curry and paprika. Bake for 30 minutes or until the vegetables are cooked.

Nutrition:

Energy (calories): 1162 kcal

Protein: 158.5 g

Fat: 46.28 g

Carbohydrates: 41.42 g

12.   Chicken And Cucumber Sandwich

Preparation time: 10 minutes

Cooking time: 25 minutesServings: 4

Ingredients:

12 pieces of chicken breast (sauce)

Cucumber slices

One red pepper

50g fresh basil

A spoon of olive oil

Tablespoon pine nuts

garlic cloves

Directions:

Wash and cut the cucumber into thin strips, then cut the pepper into small pieces.Place basil, olive oil, pine nuts, and garlic in the food processor. Mix wellAdd salt and pepper to taste if necessary.Place a piece of chicken fillet on a plate, season with a teaspoon of pesto sauce, and sprinkle cucumber and pepper on the branches.Gently roll the chicken fillet into delicious bread.If necessary, use a cocktail skewer to secure the sandwich.

Nutrition:Energy (calories): 490 kcal Protein: 32.11 g Fat: 23.88 g

Carbohydrates: 38.07 g

13.   Hazelnut Balls

Preparation time: 10 minutes

Cooking time: 25 minutes

Servings: 4

Ingredients:

Jujube 130g

140 g hazelnuts

Cocoa powder spoon

/ 2 teaspoons vanilla extract

One teaspoon of honey

Directions:

Place the hazelnuts in a food processor and grind them until hazelnut powder is obtained (of course, finished hazelnut powder can also be used).Put the hazelnut powder in a bowl and set aside.Put the date in the food processor and grind until you get a bullet.Add hazelnut powder, vanilla extract, cocoa powder, and honey and mix well.Take the food processor mixture and turn it into a beautiful ball.Place the ball in the refrigerator. Nutrition: Energy (calories): 925 kcal Protein: 20.96 g Fat: 85.06 g Carbohydrates: 30.29 g

14.   Stuffed Eggplant

Preparation time: 10 minutes

Cooking time: 45 minutes

Servings: 4

Ingredients:

eggplant

A spoon of coconut oil

Onion slices

250 grams minced meat

Clove garlic

Tomato slices

One tablespoon tomato paste

One caper manually

fresh basil by hand

Directions:

Finely chop onion and garlic. Cut the tomatoes into small pieces and chop the basil leaves.

Bring the kettle to a boil, add the eggplant and cook for about 5 minutes.

Drain the water to cool a little, and then use a spoon to remove the flesh (leaving a margin of about 1 cm on the skin). Destroy the pulp and set it aside.

Place the eggplant in the pan.

Preheat the oven to 175 ° C.

Heat 3 tablespoons of coconut oil in a pan over low heat, and then coat the onions with a layer of onions.

Add ground beef and garlic, and then fry until the beef melts.

Add chopped eggplant, tomato slices, capers, basil, tomato sauce, and fry in a covered pan for 10 minutes.

Season with salt and pepper.

Add the beef mixture to the eggplant and fry in the oven for about 20 minutes.

Nutrition:

Energy (calories): 943 kcal

Protein: 101.76 g

Fat: 8.54 g

Carbohydrates: 133.46 g

15.   Teriyaki Chicken And Cauliflower Rice

Preparation time: 20 minutes

Cooking time: 2hourd to 4hours

Servings: 4

Ingredients:

500 g chicken breast

90 ml of coconut amino acid

A spoon of coconut sugar

A scoop of olive oil

One teaspoon sesame oil

50 grams fresh ginger

Garlic clove

250 g Chinese cabbage

leek

A piece of bell pepper

Cauliflower Fried Rice)

One slice onion

One teaspoon clarified butter

50 grams fresh coriander

One lime slice

Directions:

Cut the chicken into squares: mix coconut amino acids, coconut sugar, olive oil, and sesame oil in a small bowl.

Chop ginger and garlic and add the marinade. Place the chicken in the refrigerator marinade overnight.

Finely chop Chinese cabbage, chives, garlic, and pepper, and add to slow cooker. Finally, add the marinated chicken and cook for about 2 to 4 hours.

When the chicken is almost ready, you can cut the cauliflower into florets. Then put the florets in the food processor and mix briefly to prepare the rice.

Chop the onions, heat the pan with a teaspoon of clarified butter, and then fry the onions. Then add cauliflower rice and cook it.

Sprinkle rice with chicken and cauliflower on a plate and garnish with coriander and lime wedges.

CHAPTER 3:

Dinner

16.   Mexican Stuffed Peppers

Preparation time: 10 minutes

Cooking time: 45 minutes

Servings: 4

Ingredients:

Four large bell peppers

1 lb. of ground chicken — or turkey

2 tsp. of extra virgin olive oil

1 tsp. of ground chili powder

1 tsp. of garlic powder

1 tsp. of ground cumin

½ tsp. of kosher salt

One can of fire-roasted diced tomatoes — with juices, 14 ounces

¼ tsp. of black pepper

One ¼ c. of shredded cheese — Pepper Jack, Monterey Jack, cheddar, or similar cheese, divided

1 ½ c. cooked of brown rice — cauliflower or quinoa rice

Directions:

Preheat the oven at 375 degrees F. Cover a 9x13-inch baking dishes lightly with a nonstick spray. Break the bell peppers in half from top to bottom. Remove the seeds and membranes and put the cut side in the prepared baking dish.

Heat your olive oil in a large nonstick skillet over medium-high heat. Add rice, chili powder, cumin, garlic powder, salt, and pepper to taste. Cook, boil the meat until the chicken is browned and cooked through, about 4 minutes. Drain any excess liquid, and then pour in the can of the diced tomatoes and their juices. Let it simmer for 1 minute. Remove from heat

Mix the chicken and tomatoes mix with the rice and 3/4 cup of the shredded cheese. Mount the mix as filling inside the peppers, then top with the remaining cheese.

Pour a little water into the pan with the peppers — just enough to slightly cover the plate's bottom. Bake uncovered for 25 - 35 minutes until the peppers are tender and the cheese has melted. Top with some of your favorite fixtures, and enjoy the hot weather.

Nutrition: 20 g fat, 438 calories, 32 g protein, 8 g sugars, 32 g carb, 5 g fiber.

17.   Zucchini Pizza Boats

Preparation time: 10 minutes

Cooking time: 25 minutes

Servings: 4

Ingredients:

¼ tsp. of kosher salt

Four medium zucchini

One c. of pizza sauce — or a similarly prepared marinara sauce

One ¼ c. of shredded mozzarella cheese

¼ - ½ teaspoon of crushed red pepper flakes — optional

1 tsp. of Italian seasoning

¼ c. of mini pepperoni — or regular-size pepperoni or mini turkey pepperoni, sliced into quarters

2 tsp. of chopped fresh basil or thyme

2 tsp. of freshly ground Parmesan

Directions:

Place a rack in the middle of the oven—Preheat the oven to a temperature of 375 degrees Frenheight.

Lightly powder a rimmed baking sheet or 9x13-inch nonstick baking dish.

Halve each of the zucchini lengthwise. Smoothly scrape the middle of the zucchini flesh and pulp with a small spoon or melon, leaving a margin of around 1/3 inch on all sides. Arrange the shells of the zucchini on the baking sheet. Sprinkle with salt on the inside of the zucchini.

Spoon the pizza sauce into each shell and split it equally. You might need just a little more or less depending on the size of your zucchini. Put a generous amount, but don't feel like you're going to have to fill it to the rim.

Sprinkle the mozzarella over the top and sprinkle it evenly with the Italian seasoning and the red pepper flakes (if used). Scatter the pepperoni and any other desired toppings. Most of all, sprinkles with Parmesan.

Bake for 15 - 20 minutes, until the cheese, is hot and bubbly and the courgettes are soft. If needed, transform the oven to the broiler and cook the zucchini for 2 to 3 more minutes, until the cheese becomes lightly browned. Remove from the oven and then sprinkle with the fresh basil. Serve right away.

Nutrition: 6 g fat (3 g sat) 100 calories, 7 g protein, 4 g sugars, 5 g carb, 2 g fiber

18. Creamy Gluten-Free Tomato Pasta

Preparation time: 10 minutes

Cooking time: 25 minutes

Servings: 4

Ingredients:

½ c. of diced white onion

3 Tbsp. of olive oil (divided)

1 tsp. of minced garlic

8 oz. of canned Italian stewed tomatoes (drained)

10 oz. of gluten-free pasta

¼ c. of paleo mayo

One egg yolk

Optional ½ tsp. of crushed red pepper flakes

¼ tsp. each of kosher salt & black pepper

Fresh basil and cracked pepper

Direction:

In a small pan, sauté the onions and garlic in 1 tbsp. Of olive oil until fragrant, around 2 minutes. Once they're almost done, set aside.

Cook the gluten-free pasta according to the directions in a wide pot.

Drain, rinse the pasta, and place the pasta back in the pot. Hold it on low heat.

Mix the remaining 2 tsp. Of olive oil in and blend well. Kindly blend.

In a separate tub, whisk the mayonnaise and egg yolk together. Add this mixture to the pasta pot and coat until creamy. Gently mix in the sautéed onion and garlic.

Apply the tomatoes, kosher salt, and pepper to the pasta.

Mix gently over low to medium-low heat until smooth and blended.

If you are using a cooked protein, add it here.

Put the pasta in bowls. Garnish with fresh basil and crushed chili pepper.

Nutrition: 17.1 g fat, 353 calories, 9.2 g protein, 186 mg sodium, 4.8 g sugars, 42.2 g carb, 3.7 g fiber.

19.   Honey Mustard Chicken With Brussel Sprouts

Preparation time: 10 minutes

Cooking time: 25 minutes

Servings: 4

Ingredients:

Nonstick cooking spray

2 Tbsp. of fresh lemon juice (1 lemon)

1/4 c. of plus two tablespoons extra-virgin olive oil

1 Tbsp. of Dijon mustard

1 Tbsp. of honey

1 Tbsp. of whole-grain mustard

Three garlic cloves, minced

2 lb. of bone-in, skin-on chicken thighs (I.e., four medium thighs)

Kosher salt and freshly ground black pepper

1/4 large red onion, sliced

1 1/2 lb. of Brussels sprouts, halved

Direction:

Preheat to 425 ° F in the oven. Grease a large baking sheet with the non-stick cooking spray and set aside.

In your medium bowl, whisk together 1⁄4 cup of olive oil, one tablespoon of lemon juice, Dijon mustard, whole-grain mustard, honey, and garlic. Season to taste with salt and pepper.

I am using tongs to dip the chicken thighs in the sauce and brush both sides. Place your thighs on the prepared baking sheet. Remove any remaining sauce.

In a medium bowl, also combine the Brussels sprouts with the red onion. Drizzle with the remaining 2 tsp. Of olive oil and one tablespoon of lemon juice and mix until well coated. Arrange the sprouts around the chicken on a baking sheet, making sure they're not overlapping— season to taste with salt & pepper.

Roast for 30 - 35 minutes until the chicken is golden brown with an internal temp of about 165 ° F and the Brussels sprouts are crispy. Serve yourself hot.

Nutrition:: 360 calories, 30.8 g protein, 20.1 g fat (3.6 g fat), 14.5 g carb, 6.8 g sugars, 3.7 g fiber, 350.8 mg sodium.

20. Chinese Cauliflower Fried Rice Casserole

Preparation time: 10 minutes

Cooking time: 45 minutes

Servings: 4

Ingredients:

Sesame oil for the pan

1 Tbsp. grated ginger

Optional 5 oz. diced meat (chicken or pork)

One small shallot, chopped

1 lb. stir fry vegetables

Six eggs (2 in a stir fry with four on top, soft-baked)

2 tsp. garlic, minced

A handful of mung bean sprouts, optional

Three c. cauliflower or broccoli rice (about one small to medium head of cauliflower)

¼ c. gluten-free Szechuan sauce or any gluten-free sauce of choice

2 Tbsp. beef broth (you are allowed to skip if your veggies are less starchy. The broth just gives more flavor to the casserole)

Directions:

Preheat the oven to 350 F.

Apply 1-2 tbsp. Of sesame oil to a wok or wide pan and heat to medium. If you want the meat to be included, add it here. Sauté until browned and mostly cooked (in sesame oil), then remove the meat and set aside. If you're making the vegetarian alternative, skip the meat and add the shallot, ginger, and garlic to the wok/pan and stir the ingredients until fragrant – about 2 minutes.

Next, add all the vegetables and sauce to the stir. Stir until well coated, fry for 2-3 minutes.

Combine broth and two eggs into the cauliflower or cauliflower rice. The two eggs can then be added to the stir fry or added to the mixture. Either way, it works!

Stir in the fried cauliflower rice for an additional 3-4 minutes. All in all, stir-frying does not take longer than 10 minutes.Move the wok/pan ingredients to an 8 x 11 casserole dish or a baking dish.Crack four eggs at the top of the casserole, spacing them evenly. Cover with foil and then put in the oven at 350F for 15-20 minutes or until eggs have been placed. For runny eggs, remove the casserole from the oven after 12-15 minutes of baking and cut the yolk in the middle to make a watery. Return the casserole to the oven for a further 3-5 minutes. Cool or drink immediately before freezing.Garnish with green onion, coriander, sesame seeds, and optional red pepper flakes.

Nutrition: 165 calories, 11 g protein, 8.8 g fat, 11.8 g carb, 387.4 mg sodium, 2.8 g fiber, 6.2 g sugars.

21. Aromatic Chicken Breast With Kale, Red Onion, And Salsa

Preparation Time: 10 minutes

Cooking Time: 30 minutes

Servings: 4

Ingredients

120g skinless, boneless chicken breast

2 tsp. ground turmeric

Juice of ¼ lemon

1 tbsp. extra virgin olive oil

50g kale, chopped

20g red onion, sliced

1 tsp. chopped fresh ginger

50g buckwheat

Directions:

To make the salsa, remove the tomato's eye and chop it very finely, taking care to keep as much of the liquid as possible. Mix with chili, capers, parsley, and lemon juice. You could put everything in a blender, but the result is a little different.

Heat the oven to 220°C/gas 7. Marinate the chicken breast in 1 teaspoon of turmeric, lemon juice, and a little oil. Leave for 5–10 minutes.

Heat an ovenproof frying pan until hot, then add the marinated chicken and cook for a minute or so on each side, until pale golden, then transfer to the oven (place on a baking tray if your pan isn't ovenproof) for 8–10 minutes or until cooked through. Remove from the oven, cover with foil, and leave to rest for 5 minutes before serving.

Meanwhile, cook the kale in a steamer for 5 minutes. Now fry the red onions and the ginger in a little oil. Cook until it gets soft but not colored, then add the cooked kale and fry for another minute.

Next, cook the buckwheat according to the packet instructions with the remaining teaspoon of turmeric. Serve alongside the chicken, vegetables, and salsa.

Nutrition:

Energy (calories): 300 kcal

Protein: 31.76 g

Fat: 10.18 g

Carbohydrates: 21.42 g

CHAPTER 4:

Mains

22.   Thai Prawns With Buckwheat Noodles

Preparation time: 10 minutes

Cooking time: 15minutes

Servings: 1

 Ingredients:

150g peeled king prawns

Two teaspoons soy sauce or tamari

Two teaspoons of olive oil

75g Soba (buckwheat noodles)

One clove of garlic, finely chopped

One small Thai chili, finely chopped

One teaspoon finely chopped fresh ginger

20g red onions, thinly sliced

40g green celery, thinly sliced

75g green beans, roughly chopped

50g kale, coarsely chopped

100ml chicken broth

5g lovage or green celery leaves

Directions:

Cook the buckwheat noodles according to the package insert and set aside. In the meantime, you can already heat the wok, add one teaspoon of oil and fry the prawns in it with a teaspoon of soy sauce or tamari for two to three minutes. Shrimps aside, wipe the wok.

Heat the remaining oil; fry the garlic, chili, ginger, celery, beans, kale, and red onions. Add the stock, bring to the boil, and continue cooking for two minutes. Then add the noodles and prawns, bring to the boil, and sprinkle with the celery and lovage leaves.

Nutrition:

Energy (calories): 551 kcal

Protein: 25.53 g

Fat: 22.25 g

Carbohydrates: 70.85 g

23.   Glazed Tofu With Vegetables And Buckwheat

Preparation time: 10 minutes

Cooking time: 25 minutes

Servings: 4

Ingredients:

150g tofu

One tablespoon of mirin

20g Miso paste

40g green celery stalk

35g red onion

120g courgette

One small Thai chili

One garlic clove

One small piece of ginger

50g kale

Two teaspoons sesame seeds

35g buckwheat

One teaspoon turmeric

Two teaspoons of extra virgin olive oil

One teaspoon soy sauce or tamari

Directions:

Preheat oven to 400 °.

In the meantime, mix mirin and miso. Cut the tofu in half lengthwise and divide into two triangles. Briefly marinate the tofu with the mirin/miso paste while preparing the other ingredients.

Cut the celery stalks into thin slices, the zucchini into thick rings, and the onion into thin rounds. Finely chop garlic, ginger, and chili. Coarsely chop the kale and stew or blanch briefly.

Place the marinated tofu in a small casserole dish, sprinkle with the sesame seeds and bake in the oven for approx. Fifteen minutes until the marinade has caramelized slightly.

In the meantime, cook the buckwheat according to the package instructions and add turmeric to the water.

In the meantime, heat the olive oil in a coated pan and add the celery, onion, courgette, chili, ginger, and garlic—Cook over high heat for one to two minutes to three minutes at low temperature. Add a little water as required.

Serve the glazed tofu with vegetables and buckwheat.

Nutrition:

Energy (calories): 583 kcal Protein: 34.04 g

Fat: 36.03 g Carbohydrates: 43.71 g

24.   Dal With Kale, Red Onions, And Buckwheat

Preparation time: 10 minutes

Cooking time: 40 minutes

Servings: 4

Ingredients:

One teaspoon of extra virgin olive oil

One teaspoon of mustard seeds

40g red onions, finely chopped

One clove of garlic, very finely chopped

One teaspoon very finely chopped ginger

1 Thai chili, very finely chopped

One teaspoon curry mixture

Two teaspoons turmeric

300ml vegetable broth

40g red lentils

50g kale, chopped

50ml coconut milk

50g buckwheat

Directions:

Heat oil in a pan at medium temperature and add mustard seeds. When they crack, add onion, garlic, ginger, and chili. Heat until everything is soft.

Add the curry powder and one teaspoon of turmeric, mix well.

Add the vegetable stock, bring to the boil.

Add the lentils and cook them for 25 to 30 minutes until they are ready.

Then add the kale and coconut milk and simmer for 5 minutes. The Dal is ready.

While the lentils are cooking, prepare the buckwheat.

Serve buckwheat with the dal.

Nutrition:

Energy (calories): 275 kcal

Protein: 15.05 g

Fat: 4.74 g

Carbohydrates: 47.35 g

CHAPTER 5:

Meat

25.   Sirtfood Beef

Preparation Time: 10 min.

Cooking Time: 60 minutes

Servings: 2

Ingredients:

One large beef steak

One diced potato

1 tbsp.

Extra virgin olive oil

Finely chopped parsley ½ tbsp.

One sliced red onion

Sliced kale, 1 cup

Beef stock, 150 ml

One finely chopped garlic clove

Red wine, ½ cup

1 tsp. Tomato sauce

1 tbsp. water

Corn flour 1 tsp.

Directions:

Preheat your oven to 220 °C

Boil the potatoes in a saucepan for 4-5 minutes, transfer into the oven, and roast for 30-45 with a little bit of olive oil. Turn every ten minutes so that the potatoes are roasted evenly. Pull out of the oven and add chopped parsley. Fry onions and garlic in a little bit of olive oil and add kale after a minute. Fry another two minutes until it turns soft.

Coat the meat in a thin layer of oil and fry on medium heat until it's cooked the way you like it. Remove from the pan, add the wine into the remaining oil and leave to bubble. Once the wine is reduced by half and appears thicker, you can pour into the stock and tomato sauce and bring to a boil. Add cornflour paste until you achieve the desired consistency. Serve with the steak and vegetables.

CHAPTER 6:

Sides

26. Garden Patch Sandwiches On Multigrain Bread

Preparation Time: 15 Minutes

Cooking Time: 0 Minutes

Servings: 4

Ingredients:

1pound extra-firm tofu drained and patted dry

One medium red bell pepper, finely chopped

One celery rib, finely chopped

Three green onions, minced

A quarter cup shelled sunflower seeds

A half-cup vegan mayonnaise, homemade or store-bought

A half teaspoon salt

A half teaspoon celery salt

A quarter teaspoon freshly ground black pepper

Eight slices whole grain bread

4 (1/4-inch) slices ripe tomato

Four lettuce leaves

Directions:

Grind the tofu put it in a large bowl. Add the bell pepper, celery, green onions, and sunflower seeds. Stir in the mayonnaise, salt, celery salt, and pepper and mix until well combined.

Toast the bread, if desired. Spread the mixture evenly onto four slices of the bread. Top each with a tomato slice, lettuce leaf, and the remaining bread. Chop the sandwiches diagonally in half and serve.

Nutrition: Carbohydrates 37g Protein 9g Fats 25g Calories 399

27.   Steamed Vegetables

Preparation Time: 10 minutes

Cooking Time: 15 minutes

Servings: 6

Ingredients:

½ pound carrots (peeled, cut into large pieces)

1-pound green beans (fresh, trimmed)

1 ½ pound red potato (cut in quarters)

½ teaspoon salt

½ teaspoon black pepper (ground)

1 cup of water

Directions:

Pour the water into the inner pot of your Instant Pot. Place the trivet inside the pot and set an Instant Pot steamer basket on top of the trivet.

Place the carrots, green beans, and potatoes in the steamer basket. Sprinkle the salt and ground black pepper over the top.

Secure the lid, move the valve to seal, choose the manual option, and select high pressure. Set the cooking time to five minutes.

When the cooking time is complete, let the pressure release naturally for 10 minutes, then quick release.

Remove the lid. Use oven mitts to lift the steamer basket out of the Instant Pot.

Serve as a side dish to your chicken, beef, pork, or main fish course.

Nutrition: Calories 118 Carbs 27.1g Fat 1g Protein 3.8g

CHAPTER 7:

Seafood

28. Salmon Teriyaki

Preparation time: 10 minutes

Cooking time: 60 minutes

Servings: 4

Ingredients:

For Marinade

(2) 6-7oz Salmon Fillets (skin on preferably)

2-3 tbsp. Soy Sauce / Tamari / Coconut Aminos

2 Large Cloves of Garlic

1 tsp. Sesame Oil

1/2 tsp. Black Pepper

1 tbsp. Lakanto Monk Fruit Sweetener

Lemon Zest (optional)

For Frying

1–2 tbsp. Oil for Frying

Directions:

Mix all ingredients in a bag and place the salmon fillets flat inside. Marinate for 30 minutes. Turn the load on the other side after 15 minutes to marinate evenly.

You can broil, grill, or pan-fry the salmon.

Heat the oil in a pan in low-medium heat. Pat excess marinade and place the salmon flat on the pan. Cook for 15 minutes while covering the pan with a lid. Flip the fish with a spatula after 6-7 minutes until it's done.

In the last 2-4 minutes, turn the heat on high to sear the salmon and crisp up the skin.

Turn the heat off and add some lemon juice on top

Garnish with green onions & lemon wedges (optional).

29.   Air Fryer Fish Sticks

Preparation time: 10 minutes

Cooking time: 25 minutes

Servings: 4

Ingredients:

1 lb. white fish (cod)

1/4 cup mayonnaise

2 tbsp. Dijon mustard

2 tbsp. water

Salt and pepper to taste

1 1/2 cups pork rind panko

3/4 tsp. Cajun seasoning

Directions:

With non-stick cooking spray, spray the rack of the air fryer.

Dry the fish and cut into the shape of sticks about 1 inch by 2 inches wide.

Add mayo, mustard, and water in a bowl and whisk.

Take another bowl and add the pork rinds and Cajun seasoning, and whisk. Season with salt and pepper to taste

Work with one fillet of a fish at a time. To coat the fish, dip the stick into the mayo mixture and then tap off the extra coating.

Then, dip into the pork rind mixture and mix to coat. Place on the rack of the air fryer.

Set to Air Fry at 400F and bake 5 minutes, then flip the fish sticks with tongs and bake another 5 minutes. Serve immediately.

Nutrition:

Energy (calories): 654 kcal

Protein: 81.75 g

Fat: 30.73 g

Carbohydrates: 9.12 g

CHAPTER 8:

Poultry

30.   Chicken Salad

Preparation time: 10 minutes

Cooking time: 25 minutes

Servings: 4

Ingredients

For the Buffalo chicken salad:

Two chicken breasts (225 g) peeled, boned, cut in half

Two tablespoons of hot cayenne pepper sauce (or another type of hot sauce), plus an addition depending on taste

Two tablespoons of olive oil

Two hearts of romaine lettuce, cut into 2 cm strips

Four celery stalks, finely sliced

Two carrots, roughly grated

Two fresh onions, only the green part, sliced

125 ml of blue cheese dressing, recipe to follow

For the seasoning of blue cheese

Two tablespoons mayonnaise

70 ml of partially skimmed buttermilk

70 ml low-fat white yogurt

One tablespoon of wine vinegar

½ teaspoon of sugar

35 g of chopped blue cheese

Salt and freshly ground black pepper

Directions:

For the Buffalo chicken salad:

Preheat the grid.

Place the chicken between 2 sheets of baking paper and beat it with a meat tenderizer so that it is about 2 cm thick, then cut the chicken sideways, creating 1 cm strips.

In a large bowl, add the hot sauce and oil, add the chicken and turn it over until it is well soaked. Place the chicken on a baking tray and grill until well cooked, about 4-6 minutes, turning it once.

In a large bowl, add the lettuce, celery, grated carrots, and fresh onions. Add the seasoning of blue cheese. Distribute the vegetables into four plates and arrange the chicken on each of the dishes. Serve with hot sauce on the side.

For the blue cheese dressing:

Cover a small bowl with absorbent paper folded in four. Spread the yogurt on the paper and put it in the fridge for 20 minutes to drain and firm it.

In a medium bowl, beat the buttermilk and frozen yogurt with mayonnaise until well blended. Add the vinegar and sugar and keep beating until well blended. Add the blue cheese and season with salt and pepper to taste.

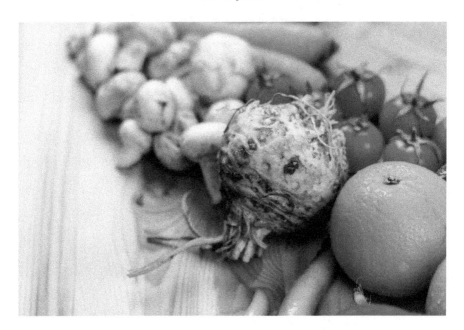

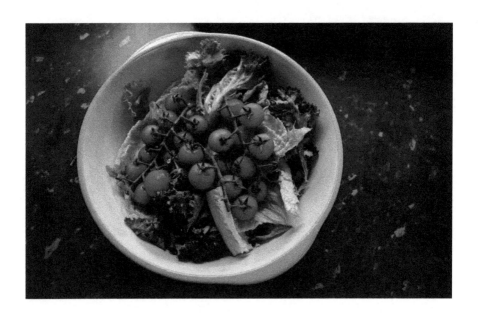

CHAPTER 9:

Vegetable

31. Cauliflower Cakes

Preparation Time: 15 minutes

Cooking time: 7 minutes

Servings: 5

Ingredients:

1 cup cauliflower, shredded

One egg, beaten

5 oz. Swiss cheese, shredded

Two tablespoons almond flour

½ teaspoon ground black pepper

¼ teaspoon salt

One tablespoon avocado oil

Directions:

Place the shredded cauliflower and beaten egg in the big bowl.

Sprinkle the ingredients with shredded cheese.

Then add almond flour, ground black pepper, and salt.

With the help of the spoon, mix up the mass well.

When it is homogenous and smooth – the cauliflower mixture is ready.

Pour avocado oil into the skillet and preheat it until it starts to boil.

Make the small cauliflower cakes with the big spoons help and place them in the hot skillet.

Press the cakes a little and roast them for 3 minutes from each side. When the cauliflower cakes get light brown color, transfer them to the plate. Dry them with a paper towel if needed.

Nutrition: calories 194, fat 14.7, fiber 1.9, carbs 5.4, protein 11.6

32. Vegetable Plate

Preparation Time: 10 minutes

Cooking time: 40 minutes

Servings: 9

Ingredients:

1/3 cup cherry tomatoes

Two bell peppers one eggplant, trimmed

One zucchini, cut 1/3 cup okra, trimmed

One tablespoon butter

One tablespoon sesame oil

One tablespoon fresh rosemary

One teaspoon salt

One teaspoon chili flakes

½ teaspoon ground nutmeg

Directions:

Slice the eggplant and zucchini roughly and transfer them to the tray.

Chop the okra roughly and add to the tray too. Then add cherry tomatoes, bell peppers, and mix up the vegetables gently with the hand palms' help. Sprinkle the vegetables with sesame oil, fresh rosemary, salt, chili flakes, ground nutmeg, and butter. Mix up the vegetables one more time. Preheat the oven to 365F.

Place the tray with the vegetables in the oven and cook for 40 minutes.

Mix up the vegetables with the help of the spatula from time to time.

Nutrition: calories 54, fat 3.1, fiber 2.8, carbs 6.6, protein 1.2

33.   Rutabaga Gratin With Spinach

Preparation Time: 10 minutes

Cooking time: 25 minutes

Servings: 4

Ingredients:

7 oz. rutabaga, sliced

4 oz. Parmesan, grated

One teaspoon ground black pepper

½ cup heavy cream

One teaspoon dried oregano

4 oz. prosciutto, sliced

One teaspoon butter

½ cup water, for cooking

Directions:

Bring the water to boil and add sliced rutabaga.

Boil it for 5 minutes over low heat.

Then drain water.

Spread the casserole mold with butter.

Place the sliced rutabaga in the casserole mold and flatten it.

Then pour heavy cream into the saucepan and bring it to boil.

Add grated Parmesan, ground black pepper, dried oregano, and stir it.

Place the sliced prosciutto over the rutabaga.

Preheat the oven to 375F.

Pour the massive cream mixture over the gratin and transfer it to the oven.

Bake gratin for 20 minutes.

Chill the cooked gratin a little before serving.

Nutrition: calories 213, fat 14.3, fiber 1.5, carbs 6.5, protein 16.1

CHAPTER 10:

Soup, Curries and Stews

34.   Chicken Stock

Preparation Time: 10 minutes

Cooking Time: 200 minutes

Servings: 4

Ingredients:

3 kg poultry bones for the rear (ideally natural)

1 tsp. salt

Three onions

300 g carrots (3 carrots)

250 g leek (1 stick)

12 dark peppercorns

Directions:

Rinse the poultry bones cold during a colander and allow them to channel.

Roughly slash the bones.

Place the bones in a huge pot, spread with approx. 4 l of water, and include salt.

Bring poultry stock to a bubble. Skim off the rising froth with a froth trowel.

Peel onions and carrots, clean and wash leeks, cut everything into enormous pieces.

After skimming, add the vegetables and peppercorns to the pan. Let it cook open for around 2 1/2 hours on low warmth, continually skimming if important. Put the poultry stock through a coarse strainer toward the finish of the cooking time and afterward through a fine one.

Chill poultry stock for the nonce and evacuate the solidified fat layer the subsequent day. Bring the poultry stock to the bubble another time, skim it and let it come right down to 1.2 l. Let cool another time. Presently it remains new within the refrigerator for as long as three days. For an extended period of usability, freeze poultry stock during a cooler sack (firmly shut!) Or within the ice 3D shape compartment. Tip: Rinse clean safeguarding containers with bubbling water, flip around them on a kitchen towel, and allow them to channel. At that time, empty the poultry stock into the boxes while bubbling hot, closes them and flips round the boxes for five minutes. The poultry stock will keep going for a few months if hand contact within the containers and tops has been maintained at a strategic distance.

35.   Chestnut Soup With Pear And Nut Topping

Preparation Time: 10 minutes

Cooking Time: 30 minutes

Servings: 4

Ingredients:

One shallot

Four parsnips

400 g chestnuts (pre-cooked; vacuumed)

2 tbsp. vegetable oil

600 ml vegetable stock

30 g hazelnut bits (2 tbsp.)

One pear

1 tsp. Nectar

½ tsp. turmeric powder

2 tbsp. squeezed orange

200 g topping

Salt

Pepper

2 stems parsley

Directions:

Peel the shallot, clean, strip, and wash the parsnips.

Cleave the shallot and one parsnip. Generally cut chestnuts.

Heat 1 tablespoon of oil in a pot. Braise shallot in it over medium warmth for two minutes, include chestnuts and parsnip pieces, and braise for 3 minutes. Pour within the stock and cook over medium heat for around a quarter-hour.

Meanwhile, dice the remainder of the parsnips—cleave hazelnuts. Wash, quarter, center, and cut the pear into blocks.

Heat the remainder of the oil during a look for gold garnish. Fry the parsnip 3D shapes for 5-7 minutes. At that time, include nuts, pears, nectar, turmeric, and squeezed orange and caramelize for two minutes over medium warmth.

Puree the soup with cream and season with salt and pepper. Wash parsley, shake dry, and cleave. Pour the fixing over the casserole and sprinkle with parsley.

Nutrition:

Energy (calories): 1764 kcal

Protein: 21.43 g

Fat: 80.84 g

Carbohydrates: 244.04 g

36.   Potato Mince Soup With Mushrooms

Preparation Time: 10 minutes

Cooking Time: 35minutes

Servings: 4

Ingredients:

600 g overwhelmingly hard-bubbled potatoes

200 g leek (1 little stick)

2 tbsp. rape oil

800 ml of vegetable stock

Salt

½ tsp. ground cumin

200 g mushrooms

400 g ground hamburger

½ tsp. dried marjoram

200 g topping

20 g parsley (0.5 bundles)

40 g pecans

Directions:

Peel, wash, and cut the potatoes into little blocks. Clean and wash the leek, divide lengthways, and dig fine rings.

Heat 1 tablespoon of rape oil during a pan, include the potatoes and, therefore, the leek, and sauté for 3-4 minutes over medium warmth. Pour within the stock, season with salt and caraway, and cook for 10-15 minutes.

Meanwhile, clean mushrooms, wash if necessary, and dig cuts. Warmth the remainder of the oil during a skillet, sauté the minced meat for five minutes while mixing; at that time, includes the mushrooms and fry for a further 3 minutes—season with marjoram, salt, and caraway.

Therefore, add the cream and the minced mushroom blend to the soup, mix, and let it heat up. Wash parsley, shake dry, and hack. Generally slash pecans. Serve soup decorated with parsley and pecans.

CHAPTER 11:

Snacks & Desserts

37.   Matcha Protein Bites

Preparation time: 10 minutes

Cooking time: 60 minutes

Servings: 12

Ingredients:

Almond butter - .25 cup

Matcha powder – 2 teaspoons

Soy protein isolate – 1 ounce

Rolled oats - .5 cup

Chia seeds – 1 tablespoon

Coconut oil – 2 teaspoons

Honey – 1 tablespoon

Sea salt - .125 teaspoon

The Directions:

In a food processor, combine all of the matcha protein bite ingredients until it forms a mixture similar to wet sand that will stick together when squished between your fingers.

Divide the mixture into twelve equal portions. You can do this by eye while estimating, or you can use a digital kitchen scale if you want the parts to be exact. Roll each portion between the palms of your hands to form balls.

Chill the bites in the fridge for up to two weeks.

Nutrition:

Energy (calories): 411 kcal

Protein: 4.39 g

Fat: 34.58 g

Carbohydrates: 32.9 g

38.   Chocolate-Covered Strawberry Trail Mix

This trail mix is excellent as it has a medley of complementary sirtfoods that will energize you throughout the day. Not only that but unlike most snacks, it can be stored at room temperature for extended lengths, making it easy to take with you anywhere you might go.

Preparation time: 15 minutes

Cooking time: 5 minutes

Servings: 10

Ingredients:

Freeze-dried strawberries – 1 cup

Dark chocolate chunks - .66 cup

Walnuts, roasted – 1 cup

Almonds, roasted - .25 cup

Cashews, roasted - .25 cup

Directions:

Mix all of the trail mix ingredients in a bowl, store it in a large glass jar, or divide each serving into its transportable plastic bag.

 Store for up to one month.

Nutrition: calorie:Energy (calories): 737 kcal Protein: 16.94 gFat: 70.04 gCarbohydrates: 23.16 g

39.   Baked Salmon Cake Balls With Rosemary Aioli

Preparation time: 5 minutes

Cooking time: 40 minutes

Number of servings: 6

Ingredients:

For salmon cake balls:

1 pound wild salmon fillets

Pepper to taste

¼ yellow bell pepper, chopped

¼ red bell pepper chopped

1/3 cup breadcrumbs

¼ cup chopped parsley

¼ cup chopped spinach

¼ cup Dijon mustard

Two tablespoons lemon juice

¼ cup vegan mayonnaise

One small egg, at room temperature

One tablespoon sriracha sauce

Two tablespoons fresh lemon juice

Salt to taste

One small red onion, chopped

½ jalapeño, diced

½ - 1 tablespoon Old Bay seasoning

For rosemary aioli

¼ cup vegan mayonnaise

One clove garlic, peeled, crushed, minced

One sprig rosemary, chopped

Salt to taste

One tablespoon fresh lemon juice

Directions:

Preheat the oven to 400°F.

Prepare a baking sheet by lining it with parchment paper.

Sprinkle salt and pepper all over the salmon and place it on the baking sheet. Place the baking sheet in the oven and roast until it flakes when pierced with a fork. It should take around 20 minutes.

Take out the baking sheet from the oven and let it cool for 5 minutes. Shred the salmon into bite-size chunks.

Combine onion, jalapeño, Old Bay seasoning, parsley, egg, lemon juice, sriracha sauce, red bell pepper, yellow bell pepper, spinach, breadcrumbs, vegan mayonnaise, and Dijon mustard in a bowl. Mix in the salmon until well combined. Divide the mixture into 12 equal portions and shape into balls. Place it on the baking sheet.

Bake for around 20 minutes or until golden brown.

Meanwhile, make the aioli by combining vegan mayonnaise, garlic, rosemary, salt, and lemon juice in a bowl.

Serve salmon balls with aioli.

Nutrition: 2 balls with one tablespoon aioli

Calories – 173 Fat – 6.7 g

Carbohydrate – 8.6 g

Protein – 20 5 g

40.   Healthy Coffee Cookies

Preparation time: 15 – 20 minutes

Cooking time: 12 - 15 minutes

Number of servings: 20

Ingredients:

For dry ingredients:

½ cup cocoa, unsweetened

Six tablespoons all-purpose flour

½ cup whole-wheat flour

¾ tablespoon finely ground coffee beans or instant coffee

½ teaspoon baking soda

¾ teaspoon ground cinnamon

¼ teaspoon kosher salt

For wet ingredients:

Three small eggs, lightly beaten

¼ cup nonfat or low-fat plain Greek yogurt

½ tablespoon olive oil

½ + 1/8 cup blueberries

½ ripe banana - ¼ cup honey

One teaspoon pure vanilla extract

¼ cup dark or semi-sweet chocolate chips

Directions:

Preheat the oven to 350°F.

Prepare a baking sheet by spraying with nonstick cooking spray. Set it aside.

Combine all the dry ingredients, i.e., whole-wheat flour, all-purpose flour, cocoa, cinnamon, salt, baking soda, and coffee, in a mixing bowl.

Place banana in a microwave-safe bowl and cook on high for about 50 seconds.

Mash the banana and add into a bowl. Also, add eggs, yogurt, oil, honey, and vanilla. Mix until well incorporated.

Pour the wet ingredients into the dry ingredients and mix until just combined, making sure not to over-mix.

Add chocolate chips and blueberries and fold gently.

Make 20 equal portions of the mixture and place it on the baking sheet. It should be approximately 1-½ tablespoons per piece.

Press the cookies lightly. You can use a fork to do so.

Place the baking sheet in the oven and bake for about 12 – 14 minutes. When the cookies are ready, they will be visibly hard around the edges.

Cool on the baking sheet for 10 minutes. Loosen the cookies by pushing a metal spatula underneath the cookies. Transfer onto a wire rack

Let it cool completely before transferring it into an airtight container.

 Nutrition: 1 cookie

Calories 60

Fat 1.5 g

Carbohydrate – 11 g

Protein 2 g

41.   Healthy Strawberry Oatmeal Bars

Preparation time: 20 minutes

Cooking time: 35 – 40 minutes

Servings: 8

Ingredients:

For strawberry bars:

½ cup old-fashioned rolled oats

Three tablespoons light brown sugar

1/8 teaspoon kosher salt

1 cup small-diced strawberries, divided

½ tablespoon fresh lemon juice

Six tablespoons white whole wheat flour

1/8 teaspoon ground ginger

Three tablespoons unsalted butter, melted

½ teaspoon cornstarch

Three teaspoons granulated sugar, divided

For the vanilla glaze: Optional

¼ cup powdered sugar sifted

½ tablespoon milk

¼ teaspoon pure vanilla extract

Directions:

Preheat the oven to 350°F.

Set the rack in the center of the oven.

Prepare a small square or rectangular baking pan by lining it with a large parchment paper sheet such that the extra sheet is hanging from 2 opposite sides.

Add oats, brown sugar, flour, salt, and ginger into a bowl and stir well.

Add butter and mix until well combined and sort of crumbly.

Take out about four tablespoons of the mixture into a bowl and set it aside.

Transfer the rest of the mixture into the baking pan. Press it well onto the bottom of the baking pan.

Spread ½ cup chopped strawberries over the crust—dust cornstarch over it.

Drizzle lemon juice over the strawberries. Sprinkle 1 ½ teaspoons sugar.

Spread remaining strawberries and 1 ½ teaspoons sugar over it.

Scatter the retained crumb mixture on top.

Place the baking dish in the oven and bake for about 30 – 35 minutes or until golden brown on top.

Take out the baking dish and place it on the wire rack to cool.

Meanwhile, make the glaze. For this, add powdered sugar, milk, and vanilla into a bowl and whisk well.

Lift the bars along with the parchment paper and place it on your cutting board.

Pour glaze on top. Cut into eight equal bars and serve.

Place leftover bars in an airtight container. Place it in the refrigerator until use. It can last for five days.

Nutrition: 1 bar without glaze

Calories 100

Fat 5 g Carbohydrate – 14 g

Protein 2 g

42.   Parsley Cheese Balls

Preparation time: 15 minutes

Cooking time: 0 minutes

Servings: 12

Ingredients:

¼ cup shredded, Kraft 2% milk sharp cheddar cheese

One package (8 ounces) Philadelphia Neufchatel cheese, softened

½ tablespoon finely chopped green onion

½ tablespoon finely chopped red pepper

¼ cup finely chopped parsley

One teaspoon Dijon mustard

Six stalks of celery cut each into four equal pieces crosswise

60 whole-wheat Ritz crackers

Directions:

Add Neufchatel and cheddar cheeses into a bowl. Beat with an electric hand mixer until well combined. Stir in green onion, red pepper, and Dijon mustard. Place the bowl in the refrigerator for an hour. Divide the mixture into 12 equal portions and shape into balls. (It should be two tablespoons cheese mixture per piece.) Place parsley on a plate. Dredge the balls in parsley. Place on a plate. Chill until use. Each serving should consist of a cheese ball with two pieces of parsley and 5 Ritz crackers.

Nutrition: 1 cheese ball + 2 pieces celery + 5 crackers

Calories – 130 Fat – 7 g

Carbohydrate – 12 g

Protein – 3 g

43.   Baked Kale Chips

Preparation time: 10 minutes

Cooking time: 10 minutes

Number of servings: 3

Ingredients:

½ bunch kale (hard stems and ribs discarded), torn into bite-size pieces

Salt to taste

½ tablespoon olive oil

Spices of your choice to taste (optional)

Directions:

Preheat the oven to 350°F.

Prepare a baking sheet by lining it with parchment paper.Dry the kale using a salad spinner. If you do not have a salad spinner, pat the leaves dry with paper towels.Place kale on the baking sheet. Trickle oil over it. Sprinkle salt over the kale and spread it evenly.Place the baking sheet in the oven and bake for about 12 – 14 minutes or until crisp.Cool completely and serve. Store the leftovers in an airtight container.

NutritionCalories 58Fat 2.8 g Carbohydrate 7.6 g Protein 2.5 g

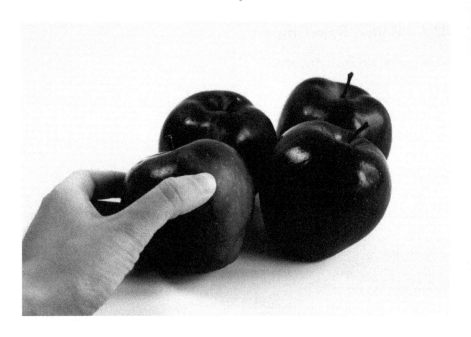

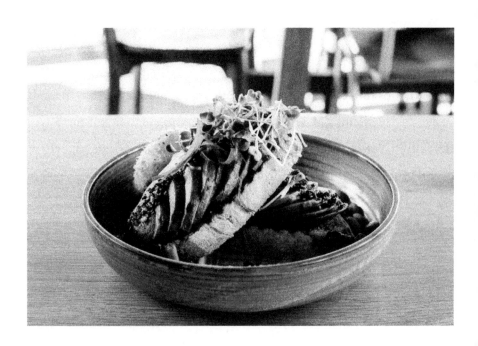

CHAPTER 12:

Desserts

44.   Matcha Green Juice

Preparation time: 10 minutes

Cooking time: 0 minutes

Total time: 10 minutes

Servings: 2

Ingredients

5 ounces fresh kale

2 ounces fresh arugula

¼ cup fresh parsley

Four celery stalks

One green apple, cored and chopped

1 (1-inch) piece fresh ginger, peeled

One lemon, peeled

½ teaspoon matcha green tea

Directions

Add all ingredients into a juicer and extract the juice according to the manufacturer's method.

Pour into two glasses and serve immediately.

Nutrition

Energy (calories): 102 kcal

Protein: 8.27 g Fat: 1.96g

Help Carbohydrates: 19.24 g

45.   Celery Juice

Preparation time: 10 minutes

Cooking time: 0 minutes

Servings: 2

Ingredients

Eight celery stalks with leaves

Two tablespoons fresh ginger, peeled

One lemon, peeled

½ cup of filtered water

Pinch of salt

Directions:

Place all the ingredients in a blender and pulse until well combined.

Through a fine mesh strainer, strain the juice and transfer it into two glasses.

Serve immediately.

Nutrition

Energy (calories): 86 kcal

Protein: 2.6 g

Fat: 6.3g Carbohydrates: 6.2 g

46.   Kale & Orange Juice

Preparation time: 10 minutes

Cooking time: 0 minutes

Servings: 2

Ingredients

Five large oranges, peeled

Two bunches of fresh kale

Directions

Add all ingredients into a juicer and extract the juice according to the manufacturer's method.

Pour into two glasses and serve immediately.

Nutrition

Calories 315

47.   Apple & Cucumber Juice

Preparation time: 10 minutes

Cooking time: 0 minutes

Servings: 2

Ingredients

Three large apples, cored and sliced

Two large cucumbers, sliced

Four celery stalks

1 (1-inch) piece fresh ginger, peeled

One lemon, peeled

Directions

Add all ingredients into a juicer and extract the juice according to the manufacturer's method. Pour into two glasses and serve immediately.

Nutrition

Energy (calories): 130 kcal

Protein: 0.91 g Fat: 0.53 g

Carbohydrates: 34.76 g

48.   Chocolate Cashew Truffles

Preparation Time: 10 minutes

Cooking Time: 35 minutes

Servings: 4

Ingredients:

1 cup ground cashews

1 tsp. of ground vanilla bean

½ cup of coconut oil

¼ cup raw honey

Two flax meal

Two hemp hearts

Two cacao powder

Directions:

Mix all the ingredients and prepare the truffles by rolling small amounts of mixture and balls. Sprinkle the coconut flakes on top.

Nutrition: Calories: 187kcal Fat: 16.5g Carbohydrate: 6g Protein: 2.3g

49.   Double Almond Raw Chocolate Tart

Preparation Time: 10 minutes

Cooking Time: 35 minutes

Servings: 4

Ingredients:

1½ cups of raw almonds

¼ cup of coconut oil, melted

One raw honey

8 oz. dark chocolate, chopped

1 cup of coconut milk

½ cup unsweetened shredded coconut

Directions:

Crust:

Chopped almonds and add melted coconut oil, raw honey, and combine. Using a spatula, spread this mixture into a cake pan.

Filling:Put the chopped chocolate in a bowl, heat the coconut milk and pour over the chocolate, and whisk.

Pour the filling into the pie shell. Refrigerate. Toast the almond flakes and sprinkle the cake.

Nutrition: Calories: 291 Fat: 9.4g Carbohydrate: 23.4g Protein: 12.4g

50.   Bounty Bars

Preparation Time: 10 minutes

Cooking Time: 35 minutes

Servings: 4

Ingredients:

2 cups desiccated coconut

Three coconut oil - melted

1 cup of coconut cream - full fat

4 of raw honey

1 tsp. ground vanilla bean

Coating:

Pinch of sea salt

½ cup cacao powder

Two raw honey

1/3 cup of coconut oil (melted)

Directions:

Combine coconut oil, coconut cream, and honey, vanilla, and salt. Pour over the dried coconut and mix well.

Shape the coconut mixture into balls and freeze. Or pour the entire mixture into a pan, freeze, and cut into bars once frozen.

Prepare the topping by mixing salt, cocoa powder, honey, and coconut oil. Dip frozen coconut balls/bars into the chocolate coating, place on a tray, and freeze again.

Nutrition: Calories: 120 Fat: 4.3g Carbohydrates: 16.7g Protein: 1g

51.   Chocolate Cream

Preparation Time: 10 minutes

Cooking Time: 35 minutes

Servings: 4

Ingredients:

One avocado

Two coconut oil

Two raw honey

Two cacao powder

1 tsp. ground vanilla bean

Pinch of salt

¼ cup almond milk

¼ cup goji berries

Directions:

Blend all the ingredients in the food processor until smooth and thick.

They are distributed in four cups, decorated with goji berries, and refrigerated overnight.

Nutrition: Calories: 200kcal Fat: 4.3g Carbohydrate: 25.2g Protein: 12.8g

Conclusions

Most diets have been proven to be just a temporary fix. If you want to keep weight off for a good while maintaining muscle mass and ensuring that your body stays healthy, then you need to be following a diet that activates your sirtuin genes: in other words, the Sirtfood Diet.

Sirtuins play an essential role in burning body fat and also help to increase the metabolic rate. But sirtuin genes aren't just responsible for weight loss and muscle gain—they also help prevent illnesses such as heart disease, diabetes, bone problems, Alzheimer's, and even cancer. To activate these genes, you must eat foods that are high in the plant-based proteins polyphenols. These are known as sirtfoods and include kale and walnuts and drinks such as green tea and red wine.

It is essential to eat a diet that combines whole, healthy, nutritious ingredients with various sirtfoods. These ingredients will all work together to increase the bioavailability of the sirtfoods even further. And there's no need to count calories: just focus on sensible portions and consume a diverse range of foods—including as many sirtfoods as you can and eating until you feel full.

You should also ensure you have a green sirtfood-rich juice every day to get all of those sirtuins- activating ingredients into your body. Also, feel free to indulge in tea, coffee, and the occasional glass of red wine. And most importantly, be adventurous. Now is the time to start leading a happy, healthy, and fat-free life without having to deprive you of delicious and satisfying food.

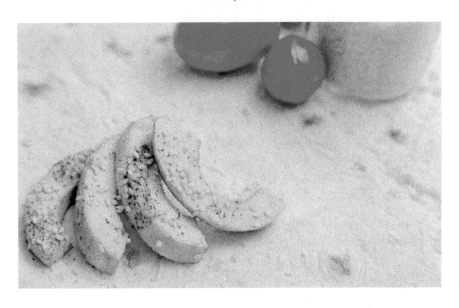

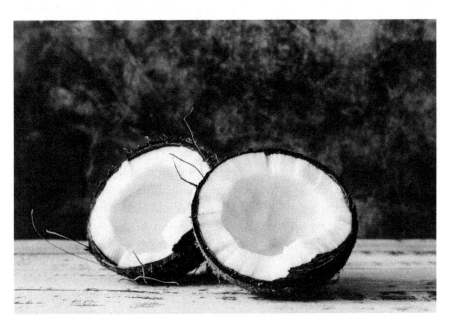